Skill, will and a healthy dose of courage

A survival guide for UK healthcare leaders

2019 EDITION

Heather Taylor MSc

For Dan

FOREWORD

Every day, tens of thousands of managers and clinical leaders pitch up to work in the UK health system determined to do a good job.

One glance at the inbox and the caffeine consumed on the morning commute feels woefully inadequate. Meetings that have mysteriously appeared overnight sit in the calendar alongside slots already booked. Texts and messages alerting to issues more pressing than the issues that are already pressing conspire to scupper the day.

Welcome to the world of healthcare leadership in the 21st century.

I have been one of those leaders. I have experienced the gut wrenching roller coaster of good, bad and dreadful moments. I've had days and weeks navigating and circumnavigating barriers and constraints.

I have pondered long and hard about how to do what's right despite the odds, and I have faced a daily battle to keep sane in a system where illogicality lurks round every corner.

The UK health system is challenged like never before, and huge numbers of incredibly loyal and dedicated staff are facing relentless pressure to stop the wheels falling from the bus.

And amongst them, managers and clinical leaders face scrutiny from every angle.

"What are you doing to keep things safe; to keep things moving; to balance the books; to improve quality?"

All roads lead to these dedicated, long suffering individuals, and getting through the day unscathed can be tough.

Switch on any news broadcast, and you will stumble upon reports of radical changes in health and social care. Talk to anyone who works in the system and they will tell you about change being the only constant in their working lives.

When I joined the UK health service, I quickly deduced that there really is no master plan.

I saw some great people do some great things in seemingly impossible situations.

I also learned that whilst regulators, patient groups, think tanks, boards, executive committees, auditors, management consultants and commissioners produce forests of documents, no-one holds all the answers.

Huge investment in initiatives to transform, re-form, better perform and dance in the storm (OK, I made the last one up), have generated some great examples of what's possible.

Meanwhile, for the most part, the system is continuing to creak, and local managers and leaders are holding things together as best they can.

These days, I have the luxury of working alongside healthcare leaders in the guise of a critical friend.

We roll our sleeves up together and fight the practical, professional and personal battles that the system throws at us.

In our quieter moments we ponder on the possibilities for radical change and indulge in thoughts of system disruption. Then the phone rings, and we land back on planet reality with an unfilled shift to fill or an (apparently) urgent paper to write.

For all its idiosyncrasies, I always find myself drawn back to healthcare because I get to work with great people who genuinely care, and who never give up.

Before we start, I should warn you that this guide is not for the faint hearted. You will find questions designed to challenge the way you work, the way you think and the way you behave.

As you dip in and out, my only plea is that you keep an open mind and respond as honestly as you can, and always remember that I challenge you from a place of empathy and with the greatest of respect.

I dedicate this survival guide to all those hardworking managers and clinical leaders who are doing their very best to keep their creaking vessels afloat.

You know who you are and I hope it helps.

Heather Taylor
May 2019

CONTENTS

- Healthcare Leadership Incompetency Framework

- Healthcare leaders' Action Avoidance Bingo

- A 'but' free day

- Re-framing the issue

- It's really not personal

- Minding your own business

- What's the point?

- Keeping it brief

CHAPTER 1
WHAT'S IN A TITLE?

I entered the world of healthcare relatively late in life. Before you leap to the conclusion that I am ancient, I simply mean that I had been around and about in the world of work for a few years before crossing the healthcare threshold.

By that time, I had worked out in the wider world with some great managers who inspired me; some who were just OK, and one or two that quite frankly I'd rather forget.

I'd also had some experience of managing staff and projects myself; learning loads as I went along, and certainly not always getting it right.

My first healthcare job was in a mid-sized hospital, and a quick glance at the staff directory showed me that healthcare leadership comes in many guises.

There were general managers, divisional managers, clinical directors, clinical leads, divisional directors, business managers, corporate managers, team leaders, co-ordinators, supervisors and many more besides.

The structures looked very complicated, but I assumed all would become clear as I took my place in a well-oiled machine.

Oh, how wrong I was!

A few months in and I had met lots of lovely, loyal and committed people, but was none the wiser about who was really supporting whom, and who had things under control.

I don't mean that there weren't clearly defined structures and formal hierarchies. There were plenty of those. It was more about me realising that I wasn't a cog in a fully functional machine at all. Rather, I seemed to be one of a growing group of people contributing blood, sweat and tears in a very complicated system that didn't make much sense. I was horrified and intrigued in equal measure.

The more time I spent in the system, the more I realised that the way everything worked (or didn't work!) was pretty much the same across the country.

Along the way, I met some great managers and leaders who had found a way to live in the shifting sands and plough on through. I also met some great teams who had somehow made sense of nonsense, and whose determination to succeed, despite everything, had won the day.

I found that there was no shortage of leadership courses to be had. I joined at a time when 'transactional' leadership was all the rage. Then came transformational, transitional, inspirational, business focussed, people focussed, money focussed.... You get the picture.

And yet, all around me, people were struggling - Struggling with relentless pressure, creaking systems and flawed processes and, not infrequently, with each other.

I went on these courses. I shared tales of woe with my peers, and returned to the coalface with bundles of handouts and dreams of a brave new world.

An hour into the first day back and I was fire fighting once again.

As time went on, it struck me that those who appeared most able to survive and thrive brought a similar combination of attributes to the table.

I pondered on these for a while, and concluded them to be:

Skill, will and a healthy dose of courage

Before assuming the role of your critical-friend, I thought I would set the tone for what lies ahead by sharing a few quick true stories from the front line.

In these stories, as they say in the movies, names have been changed to protect the innocent and any resemblance to persons living or dead is strictly co-incidental...

There was once a healthcare manager. We will call her Sadie.

Sadie told me that she absolutely 'got' what needed to be done to make her clinical service more efficient. She told me she had worked in another sector where she had successfully managed lots of complex change programmes. She also told me that she had no intention of 'ruffling feathers' with her clinical colleagues so she wouldn't actually be taking any action to drive positive change any time soon.

Sadie had plenty of textbook management skill but lacked both the will and courage to thrive in healthcare.

Another manager who we will call Sarah told me she had meticulously worked through a roster change, on paper, that she knew would be beneficial to both the service and to patients. Behind closed doors, she told me about her determination to do what was right. However, when everything was ready she backed off at the last minute - terrified of suggesting the change to her clinical colleagues. She said she would 'rather face a performance meeting with senior managers' than upset the doctors.

Sarah had both skill and will but lacked courage.

A clinical leader who we will call David told me he had some great ideas for improving his service. He told me some of these ideas and said he had no qualms about sharing them with the Board. They were ideas that were clearly going to be popular with his clinical colleagues. They were also going to be very expensive with no chance that the investment would be repaid via any tangible benefit for patients.

David had plenty of will. He was lacking in skill, and was seldom seen putting himself in a place that would test his courage.

Let's explore the title words a little more before moving on.

Skill

I was once asked to name the top three skills needed by healthcare managers and leaders.

Have a go. I don't think it's as simple as it sounds.

If you throw open this question to your colleagues, chances are that a lot more than three different words will come back at you.

If I were to ask someone not familiar with the healthcare sector to identify the top three skills they guessed were needed, I might be tempted to give them a little bit of context first:

"OK - Before coming up with the top three let me explain what you're dealing with. The person needing these skills will be working as part of a massively complex system that's been running over 70 years and that looks after over 60 million people. Despite endless restructures and re-organisations and political influence and many billions of pounds' investment, the way the system works is complicated, quite old fashioned, and sometimes, downright illogical. Over a million patients come through the doors of this system every day expecting to be helped or saved, and expecting everything to

14

run like clockwork. Some of the people you will work with have very different ideas about how things should be done, and personal interests that influence the way they behave and interact. Now name your 3 skills".

Job descriptions for healthcare leadership positions tend to include reference to general technical and professional skills, alongside general attributes and aptitudes such as 'flexibility', 'ability to influence', 'political awareness', 'horizon scanning' etc.

References to the more complicated skills necessary to survive and thrive in healthcare are less likely to feature.

For the purposes of this survival guide, I will be focussing on the skills needed to help you get through the day - Those that will help you make a positive difference despite the obstacles you will inevitably face:

Things like:

- *Nerves of steel (to face whatever the email box throws at you without tumbling into a pit of despair)*

- *The ability to keep a constant check on self-interest v service interest (even though others may not be doing the same)*

- *Ownership of a thick skin (to withstand daily battering by those more stressed than you, or those simply behaving badly)*

- *The ability to juggle double and triple booked meetings with the urgent, very urgent and even more urgent actions*

- *The ability to change the world whilst keeping it turning - during a storm*

- *The ability to switch off whilst off duty*

- *The ability to inspire, motivate, coach, coax, cajole and instruct (when appropriate)*

- *The ability to see the wood for the trees despite being in a dense forest*

- *A dark sense of humour…….*

Will

People seldom do things to the best of their ability.
They do things to the best of their willingness.
ANONYMOUS

The subject of willingness is a complex one, and I
have yet to meet a healthcare leader whose actions
haven't been influenced, to least to some degree, by
willingness (or a lack thereof).

There are many possible root causes for active
resistance. Perhaps a fear of failure, or relationship
issues clouding judgement, or a desire for self-
preservation. Worries linked to loss of power, control
or status may be at play. Self-interest may also play
a part.

Willingness, in the context of this survival guide, is
about knowing that something is the right thing to do,
and whether you tend to follow through or find
yourself digging in your heels or making excuses.

I am not suggesting for a minute that when asked to
make a difficult decision, you will be conscious that
you are resisting or refusing. I will, however,
challenge you to dig deep and consider whether

there are occasions where the person getting in the way of progress is you!

The statements that follow are paraphrased from actual conversations I have had with managers and leaders.

'Why should I (do that thing) when other's don't?'

'I don't think its part of my job actually'

'I'm not willing to make that decision?'

'Don't expect me to endorse that'

'Of course I could do that if I wanted to, but why would I do it for people who do nothing for me'.

As you read through these, I have two questions for you:

Can you hear yourself saying similar things now or in the past?

And, if you can, what do you think might have been fuelling your resistance?

Courage

Something that struck me in my early days in healthcare was how managers and leaders, at all levels, seemed reluctant to make certain types of decisions.

I don't mean life and death decisions on the front line, or in a crisis.

In fact, everyone seemed really good at leaping into action when a split second decision was needed.

It was that anything other than critical clinical decisions seemed to pass up and down layers of management, and round and round meetings, forums and committees.

I had not been working in healthcare long when I had a conversation with a respected very senior manager that shocked me.

The conversation took place at a time when hospitals were awarded star ratings to reflect external assessment of quality and safety.

The hospital he led had been awarded 2 stars out of a maximum of 3.

I remarked that this was a good starting point from which we could aspire to further improvements. He replied, in all seriousness, that I should be a little wary of aspiration. *'The middle ground is a safe place to be in healthcare',* he added. I asked what he meant and he said that he would not want to be an outlier *'in either direction'* for fear of attracting interest and attention from the national bodies.

I reflected on this exchange and found myself increasingly shocked that someone I respected so much would, effectively aspire to be average to avoid attracting too much attention to his organisation.

When I talk about the need for courage in healthcare leaders, it is really about your ability to raise your head above a parapet and challenge the status quo.

Where others are finding all excuses under the sun to leave things as they are, the courageous leader can't, and won't do that.

It's about doing what's right despite the risks; being comfortable in the knowledge that the less courageous may not follow, and weathering the storm when the waves of disruption cause people around you to act in most peculiar ways.

Pause for reflection

CHAPTER 2
MAKING SENSE OF THE MADNESS

I once had a conversation with a very senior manager who was thinking about joining the healthcare sector after an early career in banking.

Me: *You will find a lot about the system that simply doesn't make sense. This may frustrate you to the point of distraction.*

Him: *Don't worry. I'll work it out. I am sure there is a national master plan somewhere. You just haven't worked it out yet.*

His statement and attitude was arrogant and patronising.

There is no master plan. He lasted six months.

We didn't keep in touch!

From a very early age I was fascinated by how things work. I remember being about 7 when I pulled a clock apart to see what made it tick. I guess what I do now isn't much different. I'm nosey. I see something that doesn't quite work and I want to fix it.

I don't just want to be a cog.

I need to see how my cog fits in; how it adds value to the whole, and I want to step back and admire the fully functional product.

If only!

For someone inspired by engineering precision, I'm pretty amazed that I have stuck by healthcare for so long.

Actually, I'm not amazed all. The system is full of incredibly dedicated people.

If the health system were that clock I pulled apart, I would say that some of its parts are definitely past their best. Loads of extra cogs have been added over the years to bypass the ones that don't quite work. No one seems quite sure if the clock should be analogue or digital. Lots of people have had a go at winding it up. Lots of money has been invested in improving it, but not always spent on the parts that really needed it.... I could go on.

Suffice to say all of this has turned the clock into a clunky and complicated beast. And yet, somehow, by sheer determination (and a fair wind) it keeps on ticking.

This book is not about politics, so I must lay aside my theories of root cause. I will, however, be so bold as to suggest that evidence of things not joining up is everywhere you look.

Whilst I am at a point in my life where I have put in the seven day working weeks, and now try to separate work and life, I must admit that when conversations with friends and family turn to healthcare, I can't help but draw on my knowledge of the system to analyse their experiences.

Recently, an elderly relative was worried out of his mind because he had received a completely unexpected letter about a 'heart test'.

The letter gave a choice of venues to choose for the appointment including his local community health centre and two hospitals he knew had 'special heart departments'.

Needless to say, the only words that leapt from the page were 'heart' and the names of the 'specialist' hospitals.

He was convinced that a serious heart problem had somehow been detected from his routine diabetes blood test and that open-heart surgery beckoned.

I told him that in all likelihood it was an initiative from his GP's surgery where people of a certain age with certain risk factors were being given opportunities for preventative testing.

I explained that the health service is trying to keep people well these days rather than just help the ones that are actually sick.

Suitably relieved he set about sorting the appointment, not realising the possibility that admin departments may not be talking to other admin departments.

I will cut a long story very short.

Call to GP surgery: No one seemed to know why he had received a letter and what it was all about. Receptionist suggested he rang the number on the letter. Number on letter got through to answer phone suggesting he phoned his GP. Different receptionist at GPs' surgery suggested he phoned the booking department of his preferred choice directly. Booking office of preferred choice hospital had no idea what the letter was about and suggested he scanned it and emailed it over.

He is 83. He has no idea how to work a scanner. He gave up and heard nothing more about it.

I think we all have personal tales like that that we could tell.

Whilst system illogicality is all around us, I firmly believe that it's the people working within it who hold the key to returning at least some level of sanity.

Easier said than done, I know, and when you work in a world where little makes sense, even the most logical amongst us can be drawn in.

A few years ago, I was working in a hospital that had been recognised nationally for their approach to pre-operative patient assessment. I was really keen to find out what they'd done and what the impact had been.

I was introduced to a delightful and passionate doctor who had pioneered the process and delivered it by working hand in hand with her nursing and administrative colleagues.

You could see immediately why this team would impress judges in any 'Inter-professional Working' award category.

You could also see immediately how her passion to do the right thing had motivated her and her team to make a real difference.

I asked her what they had done.

She explained that before the project, the processes for pre-operative assessment had been patchy, at best. There had been different approaches taken in different clinics. Across the hospital, too many patients were coming in on the day of surgery unable to have their operations, as the necessary checks hadn't been made in time.

A massive transformation had been achieved. A multidisciplinary pre-op assessment unit had been set up. In a majority of cases, patients were able to attend the unit at the same time as being listed for surgery at their outpatient appointments.

Patients were very satisfied with the service.

Some concerns had been raised by clinicians about the risks of assessment undertaken too early; in particular where patients may acquire infections or other health problems close to the date of surgery.

Whilst recognised as a factor, there was a broad view that streamlining the process and setting up the unit was a positive move.

And then I asked the million-dollar question.

'What impact has it had on cancelled operations?'

The doctor was silent. There was a very long pause.

She finally replied.

'We haven't actually measured that to be honest'.

In another example, a Human Resources department reported national recognition of their work in capturing diversity information as part of their recruitment process.

Whilst most organisations I work with have caught up with this now, the organisation in question was hailed as a front-runner in this regard.

I asked them what their measure of success for this process was.

The manager looked at me very quizzically.

I asked if, for example, the data had been helpful in identifying the extent to which the workforce mirrored the diversity of the local community, or whether the information was helping them target under represented groups?

She replied with these exact words.

'We won a national award for our process. No one has asked us these questions before. The process is brilliant'.

Staying with HR, I spent some time working in a hospital that was struggling to attract administrative staff with the right skills and attitude for the organisation.

I met the recruitment manager and he explained to me how proud he was of the recruitment process and his surprise that it wasn't having the desired results.

I arranged for the recruitment manager to go along to observe some interviews in a business renowned for attracting, and retaining, great candidates.

Before attending the external interviews, the manager took me through the existing selection process in minute detail. He showed me extremely detailed Job Descriptions and Person Specifications.

He stressed how important it was for managers to engage in the process of writing every tiny detail of what each job entailed into the Job Profiles.

He showed me the detailed matrix managers complete at interview to match each part of the job description with an assessment of the candidate's skills and experience. He said he was shocked that despite all this, his organisation seemed to be recruiting *'masses of staff with the wrong attitude'.*

The day of him attending the external company interviews came and went. I heard nothing back so I waited a couple of days and called him.

Me: *How did it go at the interviews?*

Him: *It was complete rubbish.*

Me: *Oh, OK. - In what way?*

Him: *The interviewers only wrote really brief notes.*

Me: *Oh, OK. Is that all? What did you think of the quality of questions they were asking?*

Him: *I didn't really notice that. I was shocked they didn't have all the questions written down though.*

Me: *Oh, OK. But did they ask all the candidates the same questions?*

Him: *Yes, I think so.*

Me: *Did you take anything positive from the experience at all.*

Him: *Not really. Nice sandwiches though.*

Me: *It's a tricky one this. If you visit the company, you'd find that their staff all have a great attitude. Something must be working.*

One more example before we move on.

This one made me really sad.

A clinical team was under extreme pressure to hit a national target for routine outpatient waiting times. The target was based on a very specific group of patients who were waiting following a referral directly from their GP.

Amongst a huge pile of referral letters due for processing were some with earlier initial referral dates.

As the administrators worked through the letters to arrange appointments, I saw them put some of the letters with earlier dates back to the bottom of the pile.

I questioned why this was happening and was shocked by the response.

One of the administrators told me that their manager had instructed them to deal with the letters that would impact the target first.

This meant that each day, letters relating to patients whose appointments wouldn't impact the target would rise up the pile, only to be put back to the bottom again.

Each one of these letters represented a patient who was at home assuming their letter was progressing through a fair system towards a hospital appointment.

These administrators were good people. They knew what they were doing didn't feel right, but they were under strict instructions to deal with the letters in a certain way. None of them felt it was their place to challenge the process.

The story has a positive ending. A new manager was appointed. He was courageous. He challenged the morality of the target-focused approach; sorted the backlog, and introduced a new process that ensured both fairness and compliance.

I have concluded that there is something about the system that allows intelligent, passionate people to pursue a path of multiple processes with very little regard to outcome.

I've spent many a long hour pondering the root cause and concluded that we probably need to accept, as a given, that the healthcare system has evolved to be so overcomplicated that this type of madness can masquerade as the norm.

Some time ago, conscious that I could unwittingly blend into acceptance of odd norms, I made a promise to myself. I committed to constantly questioning if I am being drawn into the illusion that process trumps outcome.

I guess it's easy for me, as someone who gets to flit from organisation to organisation, but I firmly believe that asking this question of yourself a few times a day can be an extremely valuable discipline to adopt.

In the exercise that follows, I challenge you to reflect on your own willingness and courage to cut through the nonsense and progress things that matter.

All the scenarios below are based on real situations I have encountered.

My question to you is whether you believe that you would take action or accept the status quo.

TAKE ACTION OR LEAVE IT ALONE?

1. An administrative process has been in place for years and everyone is used to it but you know that in this era of technology there must be a better way of doing it.

2. A member of your team is quite clearly not contributing as much as the others and you know this is making people annoyed.

3. The phone number on some of the letters going out from your service is printed on letter headed paper that is out of date. You're worried you are missing some calls as a result.

4. A colleague has been absent from work a number of times and you suspect the reasons being given may be dishonest.

5. You're not convinced that a process you have introduced in your department is having the desired effect.

6. You know that the way you are buying equipment is the most expensive way.

7. A senior manager is showing favouritism to one of your staff and you believe it to be inappropriate.

8. You're regularly leaving work over two hours late and are not able to switch off on days off.

I'm guessing that if you're doing this exercise in the comfort of your home, your logical brain may have kicked in and your instinct would be to do something?

I guess the real challenge would be if you were faced with those things in real time in the workplace.

Is there a risk that you could be so wrapped up in the stresses and pressures of the day that you might unwittingly contribute to maintaining the status quo?

Don't worry.

That question is rhetorical.

Pause for reflection

CHAPTER 3
SURVIVAL

I vividly remember my first day as an NHS operational manager. I'd fancied a change and found myself volunteering for a sideways move from the relative tranquillity of a corporate office to a manic front-line management role.

Two hours in and I was told the patient booking system was down. I had two angry consultants at my door, an email inbox bursting at the seams and my shiny new bleep was flashing away like there was no tomorrow.

I asked a fellow ops manager if this was a normal day.

She replied *'Welcome to the world of NHS management. We sink or swim. We go to the pub, and we come back to sink or swim again.'*

I've been an ops manager in other sectors and couldn't help thinking that these managers weren't really being employed to manage operations, but to trouble-shoot in a system where nothing works quite like it should.

The consultants at my door were angry for a reason. The computer system was down for a reason. And the endless people bleeping me were clearly minded to bleep the manager rather than make decisions.

For the 7 year old in me who wanted to rip open the clock to see how it worked, this was all very fascinating.

For the grown up who had unwittingly found herself in the job, it was totally exhausting!

In the sections that follow I will draw on both my working experience and my subsequent learning from some wonderful (and less than wonderful) managers and leaders to offer challenges and tips to support your day-to-day survival.

Navigating the hierarchy

Personally, while I recognise the need for effective governance and lines of responsibility, I am not a great one for hierarchy for its own sake. By this, I mean I struggle with the idea of management roles that don't add any real value other than keeping tabs on the next level 'down'.

For all the movement towards *clinical leadership, local freedom* and *flat structures* I still find that most healthcare leaders are able to point to one or more people they would refer to as their 'boss'.

Of course, if you are right at the top of the tree, these 'bosses' may be external to your organisation. None the less, there will likely be individuals holding you to account, one way or the other.

If you are lucky, they will also be watching your back too.

Bosses come in all shapes, sizes and guises. There are those that are great, good, bad, plain evil and anything in between. When I joined the NHS, I found the chains of command quite fascinating - and more than a little bit odd. For a start, I had never before worked in an environment where managers' diaries were crammed with meetings with other managers, and sometimes their managers' managers.

I wasn't used to managers saying things like *'How am I meant to know what to do if my manager is always too busy to see me?'* or *'My manager has no idea what I do so isn't helpful',* or *'It's probably my manager rather than me that you need to talk to.'*

I soon learned that a lot of this stems from there being complicated lines of clinical and non-clinical accountability.

I discovered structure charts with lots of dotted lines on them, with no one quite sure who is really accountable to whom *'since the last re-structure'.*

My early experience in the NHS taught me that it's worth investing some time and energy into building a positive working relationship with your boss(es) for the sake of your health and sanity, and to ensure you can perform at your best. I have learned that provided you and your boss(es) are decent, reasonable and rational human beings, there is a ray of hope in this regard !

Everyone has good and bad days, and learning how to recognise these in each other can be extremely valuable. You can find out what strengths each of you bring to the table and use these to support each other in times of need.

Whilst stress and pressure can make people behave in the most peculiar ways, I have to say that a vast majority of managers and leaders I come across in the NHS fall into the decent and rational human being category.

Of course, I've met a few that don't, and there will be more about those later.

Healthcare leaders come from all walks of life. They exhibit traits from the full spectrum of personality preference and, for the most part, share a desire to do what's right.

When struggling with hitting targets, getting the money to stack up and doing what's best for patients, things can get extremely tense.

At times like these, it's easy for managers and leaders to blame the next tier up or down. When tempted to do this, it's sometimes helpful to step back, if only for a minute, and remember you're all in it together.

It's not about you. It's about the task in hand.

When faced with a tough decision or challenge, each layer of management and leadership needs to bring unique skills and expertise and add value to the whole.

If you fear being reprimanded, or are tempted to reprimand to deflect blame, why not take a deep breath and say.

'I don't have the answer to this one. How can we solve this together?'

In work (and life) situations where I feel things getting fractious, and where my instinct is to deflect blame, I try really hard to pause for just a second and to ask myself:

'Hang on. What part am I actually playing in resolving this?'

I genuinely believe that if we all asked ourselves this question regularly, we may sometimes be surprised at the answer. I have certainly caught myself out with this question.

For example I've had to admit to myself (on occasion), that I am not adding that much value at all; that I am getting in the way of progress because I am protecting myself or a particular colleague, or that I am falling into the trap of allowing something to be delayed to avoid action that will take courage.

Where you are finding relationships within the hierarchy tricky, it's really important not to allow the situation to escalate to such a degree that it is affecting your ability to be yourself; give of your best or get in the way of life and health. You owe it to yourself and to your organisation to take an objective look at what is going on; to take a deep breath, and to tackle it.

I do occasionally meet a manager or leader who enjoys the intrigue of complex or dysfunctional working relationships. I will dare to suggest that this can never be right, as it is, at best, a distraction to the job in hand. At worst, it ripples out to the wider team to create a fog of mistrust and toxicity.
Look out for this behaviour in yourself and others, and please don't ever fuel or encourage it.

If you have put yourself forward for a healthcare management role, it is fair to say that you can expect work to be full of challenges, and some significant frustrations.

With the best will in the world, the system itself is far from perfect. Links between organisations can be very disjointed, and I often hear colleagues talking about *perverse system-incentives, conflicting demands,* and *silo thinking.*

In your own organisation, managers at all levels will inevitably be struggling with these external things themselves so may need you to switch priorities, or to respond to ever changing sands.

If you are able to accept, as a given, that you are working within an imperfect world, there is every chance that you will be able to form a reasonable, mutually supportive relationship with your boss(es).

Bosses behaving badly

In the section above, I touched on the subject of managers who don't fall into the decent, rational category.

I believe that despite first impressions, it is always best to look for the good in people and to navigate a positive path through allowable weakness. I also believe that it is prudent to look out for signs of behaviour that might be fall outside the limits of fair or appropriate.

I am talking, here, about behaviour towards you that makes you uncomfortable, or has no rational basis. I am talking about behaviour that may indicate prejudice, bullying or harassment.

Before joining healthcare, I worked, for a while, in another part of the public sector. I started as a personal assistant and rose through the ranks to a middle management position.

My role reported into a Director.

The Director had a Deputy who clearly believed the more senior role should belong to her. She could often be found telling anyone who would listen how 'out of his depth' the Director was, and how she would do things differently if she were in charge. He was actually a perfectly competent, straightforward and reasonable boss.

As my time in my role progressed, I found her taking an increasing interest in my work and my life. She seemed very intrigued by the fact that I have never passed my driving test (long boring story!), and colleagues told me that she would quiz them about whether they found driving me to off-site meetings (that they were also attending) irritating.

I thought this was odd but thought little of it, until she called me up to her office one day to say that a number of colleagues had approached her and expressed concern about me not having a car and 'relying on them' for lifts to meetings. I knew this was quite ridiculous, but rather than challenge her, I left feeling that perhaps what she was saying was true and that my colleagues were being less than open with me.

Odd incidents like this continued for some time, and whilst I had neither the will nor courage to challenge it, I found myself getting increasingly uncomfortable in her presence. She started to take every opportunity to undermine me in meetings and to blatantly take credit for my work with a sideways glance, as if looking for a reaction.

At the time I had no idea I was being bullied and I pride myself in maintaining my dignity throughout every encounter with her. What I do know now is that she dented my confidence for a long, long time and if I could turn back the clock, I would have called time on her behaviour a lot earlier.

In another organisation, colleagues warned me that a particular senior manager had a reputation for surrounding herself by people who were good at what they did, but not too good. They warned me that she could flip from supportive to vitriolic if she felt her place as Queen Bee was challenged.

I can hear myself now saying *'Thank you for the advice, but I can't see that happening to me'*.

I think I genuinely believed that I would see it coming, and, in any event, this leader was being fine to me at the time, so maybe their fears were ill founded or based on here say.

Fast forward three months and I was being praised by a group of colleagues for a presentation I had given. Behind my back, I distinctly heard *'She's only presenting what we already know'*. I let this one go.

I'm actually pretty objective where work is concerned, and while I thought it was an odd aside from someone in her position, it was fine. And then, it got worse and worse. Exclusion from meeting invite lists. Exclusion from shared jokes in the office. I would walk into the office and everything would go quiet. And then the veiled accusations started. *'We heard through the grapevine you've been saying xxx - is this true?'*.

These were always ridiculous things that I would never say. But, as a result, peers who had once valued my input or sought my advice stopped coming to me.

Whilst the root cause of these examples was likely fragile egos, (or sociopathic tendencies), the way it manifested itself crossed the barrier of acceptable weakness.

For the sake of health and sanity, if you realise that your own behaviour, or the behaviour of people around you, isn't healthy, or is getting in the way of doing what's right, you have two choices. You can ignore it and carry on regardless (lack of will or courage perhaps?) or you can take a deep, courageous breath and start to tackle it.

I advise the latter – every time.

Boardroom behaviour

The boardroom is arguably the place where the highest levels of skill, will and courage need to be applied. It's great when it is and potentially disastrous when its not.

While it pains me to say this, I have seen deficits in one of more of these attributes play out in boardrooms far and wide.

Specifically, I have seen very senior managers around tables engaging in a game I have termed *Responsibility Ping-Pong.* It's a fascinating ritual to watch. It can be an extremely sophisticated means of deflecting attention away from critical decision-making, or to avoid individual and collective responsibility.

In the best organisations I have had the pleasure to work in, the dialogue at senior level has been open, honest, and focussed on doing what is right for patients, clients or the organisation.

These are the teams who are unafraid of debating differences of opinion behind closed doors; where everyone feels ready, willing and able to contribute their ideas and where decisions come from proper consideration of all views.

Conversely, I have seen bullying, sulking, inter-professional rivalry, disrespect, blame, buck passing, rudeness, and passive-aggression. The list goes on. These behaviours can often be concealed beneath a thin veil of pleasantry, but are nonetheless palpable and highly toxic when present.

I once worked with a senior management team who seemed pretty friendly on the surface. However, just a tiny scratch revealed some quite appalling behaviour that played out, most vividly, in the boardroom. This was a place where *Responsibility Ping-Pong* played out for all to see.

'*Why are our finances in such a mess?*' asked a non-executive director.

'*Because doctors cost too much*', said the senior nurse.

'*Yes I'd be keen to know the answer. Ask the Finance Director*' said the CEO.

'*Ask the Chief Operating Officer*' said the Finance Director.

'*Nursing is the problem*' said the Medical Director.

This is, of course, paraphrased, but you get the picture. Similar conversations played round and round in a loop to cover all subjects from patient safety to car parking charges - and anything in between.

Perhaps, most alarming in this particular scenario was the tendency of the CEO to align with the non-executive directors whilst quickly pointing the finger of blame towards colleagues.

Not surprisingly, the Executive Directors in this organisation didn't tend to stay long.

In more than one organisation, I have witnessed inappropriate senior management behaviour which has left me questioning exactly what value certain individuals were bringing to the table other than a tendency to undermine, find fault, and score points against colleagues.

More than once in these situations, I have held back from shouting

'Well done - You have succeeded in finding a misplaced semi colon in this report. Do you have anything helpful to contribute about the wider content',
or

'Well done - You have succeeded in making the person you are talking to feel three centimetres tall. Now do you have anything to say that might helpfully move this subject forward?'.

I must add that these are not daily occurrences, but certainly not infrequent.

I once worked alongside a senior management team with an operational Director who believed he should be in charge. I often wished I had recorded his behaviour in the boardroom as a teaching aid for aspiring leaders which I would call 'How not to lead'.

Specifically, if anyone spoke, he would likely roll his eyes, or sigh. He possessed an unflinching belief that his intellect was infinitely superior to everyone around him. He was bright, but also blind sighted to the fact that his desire to have both the first and last word (and all words in between) resulted in him quite regularly spouting nonsense.

All of this would have been fine had I not inadvertently allowed myself to get caught up in the hype that surrounded him. He was such a pain when challenged, that I found myself increasingly inclined to accept what he was saying. That way, I could avoid being patronised to within an inch of my life.

Encounters with him could be shorter, and working days not quite so torturous if I allowed him to believe he was right.

This experience did not damage me personally, but I reflect on this time as a period when I added considerably less value than I might have done had I been prepared to put a foot or two down, and to encourage my colleagues to do the same.

So if your become aware that an ego has landed around your top-table, so to speak, please try and be wise to this early, stick to your guns, and do what's right.

Getting on with colleagues

Alongside the relatively small number of MBAs, the fresh-faced business graduates and management trainees, I come across far more healthcare managers and clinical leaders who have risen through the ranks of their professions. It is not unusual to find people managing those who they trained with, or who once taught them.
Some of the relationships go way back, with managers now leading those with whom they once shared their deepest hopes and fears as students or trainees.

Not everyone falls into management roles willingly or wittingly. I sometimes joke that clinical directors tend to be doctors who have failed to hide quickly enough when the appointment process came round.

This is a sweeping generalisation, of course, and I have come across clinical leaders motivated to make positive changes; those keen to make a name for themselves and those looking to expand their career options.

For some clinical managers, there can be personal struggles between the desire to lead and the pull to retain some clinical work, to defend their profession and to defend ex-peers. Clinical managers can be perceived as poacher turned gamekeeper; referred to as 'joining the dark side' or treated with suspicion or mistrust.

Then there's the managers who come through the ranks of admin, or who always intended to be managers, who face a daily battle between management and leadership theory and the reality on the ground.

Regardless of their path to leadership, all healthcare leaders find themselves thrown into a world where all roads lead to them, and where pressure to deliver, in a limited time, can be intense.

I think for me, one of the first lessons I learned was to accept that however good your skills, and however worthy your intentions, there will be times when whatever you do, your colleagues will cast you in the role of 'evil manager' or 'manifestation of everything that's wrong with the system'. This is because you will often be the one charged with delivering news of what can't be done / afforded / achieved.

As a hospital manager, for example, you can't magic extra offices or consulting rooms; you can't ride roughshod over a financial bidding process; you can't provide locum staff to fill gaps if they simply don't exist, and you can't shake money from an empty tree.

Meanwhile your colleagues battling at the front line may fail to recognise the battles you are fighting behind the scenes – casting you in the role of villain without so much as a second glance.

I believe you stand the best chance of surviving all this if you can offer empathy and understanding where appropriate; be honest and transparent about the challenges and constraints you are working through and resisting the urge to blame anyone at all.

I was recently asked to support an operational manager who was having great difficulty with one of his consultant colleagues. I spoke to both parties separately. There was little love lost between them. The conversations went something like this.

Consultant about manager: To be frank, the man is stupid. He has no idea what pressure we're under. I would like to see him stop by once in a while and see what its like to deal with the chaos in clinic that he has caused. How would he feel if he were trying to see patients and had me breathing down his neck to spend less time with them. I'm guessing he goes home at night long before I do.'

Manager about consultant: To be frank, the man is a nightmare. He has no idea what pressure we're under. I would like to see him stop by once in a while and see what its like to deal with the chaos in clinic that the system has caused. How would he feel if he were trying to fix the system and had me breathing down his neck that I don't care. I'm guessing he goes home at night long before I do.

These two people were feeling similar pain from a different perspective. I suggested that the three of us met in the same room, at the same time and got replies to the prospect, as follows:

Consultant: *Complete waste of time but OK, if you're telling me I have to.*

Manager: *I'll do it but I doubt it will make any difference. I'm not likely to sleep the night before.*

We met.

I did little more than ask them to repeat what they had told me.

It went very well.

We overran our time slot and they went off to the canteen to continue the discussion 1:1. These were two decent rational people who had the courage to break ice, listen and start again.

Change and uncertainty

Excuse me while I state the obvious. The only thing constant in healthcare management is change.

It's really quite tricky to write this section without straying into the realms of big and small 'p' politics, but I will resist.

Suffice to say that in my experience, every word from a government department or regulator's pen sets forth a chain reaction that propels healthcare managers into a tailspin of frantic activity.

And then, as the chaos gives way to calm, we create action plans, more action plans and yet more action plans.

I have come across leaders who appear to thrive on the chaos and uncertainty, and others who find it deeply uncomfortable.

Change is inherently unsettling, so I will admit that I can be a little sceptical when meeting managers who appear keen to wax lyrical about their love for it. I have certainly met managers whose positivity about change gives them a reason (or, dare I say, excuse) for not driving forward actions already underway. These are those people who say *'I'm fine with things around us always being in a state of flux. It means we never actually change anything, so we actually get to do things just like we always have, to be honest.'*

Then there are those who soldier on in the knowledge that talk-about-change rarely translates to actual-change. Those who say *'I've been around the system long enough to know that initiatives come and go and come round again every few years.'*

Then there are the individuals for whom change is deeply uncomfortable and who struggle into work day after day with a steely focus on the here and now. Their fear manifests as an arms-crossed defence of the status quo. *'We've tried that before'* they cry, *'Its best to keep doing things the way we always have'*. *'It's a stupid idea'*.

There are many in between, but experience has shown me that something about the complex multiple layered healthcare system allows managers and clinical leaders to carry on regardless; seeing change as something that someone else wants, and expressing cynical views about the chance of success. There are, of course, exceptions to this. Brilliant managers and leaders who get-it, and who are able and inclined to motivate colleagues to see a new point of view, and to re-focus time and effort.

As managers and clinical leaders, you don't just have to manage your own reaction to change and uncertainty. You are also charged with managing the fears, concerns and reactions of staff affected by it.

This can be exhausting, and a place where will and courage can give way to a tendency to side with those most resistant, with cries of *'I don't want to make the changes either. It's someone else'*.

For those of you struggling with initiative fatigue, and difficulty summoning the energy to drive positive change for the greater good, it can be helpful to attack the challenge from a different angle.

To illustrate this, I will share two true stories of triumph over cynicism.

In the first, it was 2008, and hospitals were facing increasing pressure to balance their books.
At that time, there weren't caps on agency pay rates, and many hospitals had identified the subject of 'reducing nurse agency spend' as a potential source of savings. I observed hospitals tackling this issue in a number of different ways.

Senior management teams setting reduction targets and chastising their managers for failing to achieve them.

Senior management teams bringing in management consultants to diagnose the extent of the 'problem' or 'opportunity', then presenting findings to their Boards, telling their managers to deal with it and chastising them for failing.

Nursing Directors presenting the challenge to their Boards and defending the cost pressure.

Finance Directors presenting the challenge to their Boards and blaming the nursing Directors for the issue.

Nursing Directors blaming Recruitment Directors and Recruitment Directors blaming external parties.

I could go on but I'm sure you get the picture.

I received a call from a hospital hoping to resolve the issue and needing the support of an external party to 'diagnose the extent of the issue'.

My reply was to advise them not to spend any money diagnosing the problem.

I said that the extent of the issue could be determined extremely quickly using data they already had and spending five minutes with a calculator.

A conversation started, I explained that knowing the extent of the problem would be a great start and that the most powerful way to crack the issue would be to work with the nurses to resolve it.

Fast forward two weeks and I am invited to meet two of the hospital's most senior nurses. I walk in to be greeted by tightly crossed arms and glum faces.

I had no idea what they had been told about the meeting but it was clear from the outset that they had been summoned to similar sessions before.

I guessed that they had previously had many so called 'experts' paraded before them who had no idea about the pressures they faced and who were there to tell them how to do their jobs.

The conversation went something like this.

Introductions.

'I'm guessing you think I'm here to tell you what needs doing? That would actually be ridiculous, because I don't yet know what the problem is. I mean, I know your senior managers are seeing loads of money being spent on agency staff, and I'm guessing you're the best people to know why its happening. So shall we start there?'

I promise you it took very little more than that to melt the ice-cap atmosphere. The arms uncrossed, the faces lit up, and 30 minutes into an extremely positive meeting we were pretty close to root cause, and what we could do together to crack the challenge.

These nurse leaders were fantastic. We worked together for six months; playing to our respective strengths to fix what was broken and to bring folks with us. These leaders worked with their colleagues to drive agency use from hundreds of shifts a month to single figures.

On the day we got to zero shifts, we had cake!

I learned later that I was the fourth person bought in to 'sort' this problem. I guess the difference was that I didn't actually bowl in to solve it. I came in to first get to grips with exactly what needed sorting; who was best equipped to sort it, and to be everything they needed me to be while they set about fixing it.

For me, the best possible thing about this is that those who have solved the issue get to own the success and to sustain it long after I've gone. I tend to keep in touch for a while, just in case, and am seldom disappointed.

My second story features a much maligned and misunderstood group of staff whose day-to-day work was constantly criticised by hospital senior managers.

I attended a hospital management meeting where the subject of meeting patient waiting list targets was being discussed.

After a robust round of *responsibility ping pong,* most people present were keen to end the debate and were engaging in a manoeuvre which I have termed *blame an absent party.* The term is pretty self-explanatory. I challenge you to watch this play out in the meetings you attend and, if you know it's happening, to stop it in its tracks.

On this particular day, I witnessed a particularly unpleasant example of the manoeuvre as a group of very senior managers, who, quite frankly, should know better, turned their attention to a very junior group of booking assistants.

'It's the call centre staff' said a senior manager.

Seeing an opportunity to deflect blame, there was a palpable rise in energy around the room.

'Yes. They don't see how important it is to get through the bookings'.
'They keep people waiting till they hang up'

'They make mistakes'

'I heard that over half the calls are aborted. It's disgusting'.

And so it continued.

Shockingly, not one of the managers present rose to the defence of the staff. It was clear something needed to be done and I suggested it might be helpful to find out from the staff whether they felt things were fine, or whether things needed to change.

An hour later, and I was in a dingy porta-cabin across the hospital car park. I ventured into the call centre room to be greeted by a frazzled supervisor who was extremely glad to see me. *'No-one ever comes over here'* she said. *'We're hoping you might be the first person to listen to us'.*

She led me past a mountain of paper towards a group of desks where call handlers were making outgoing phone calls without so much as a breath in between. Meanwhile, the incoming phone lines were ringing and not being answered.

While the staff continued to make their calls, the supervisor took small batches of letters from the paper mountain to add to the piles already on each of the desks. I was told that these were the appointment letters and that the staff manning the phones had to get through huge quantities every day to ensure targets were met.

In order for me to understand the issues that were leading to management perception of an ineffective operation, I had arranged for a 45 minute break in outgoing calls to give the staff a chance to air their views.

The minute this time started, there was a mass exodus of staff. The supervisor said that I should excuse this as they would be taking the opportunity to go to the bathroom, as there was rarely time for a break during the shift.

When the staff returned we got down to business and we were only minutes into the discussion before the root cause and potential solutions were surfaced.

It transpired that the staff knew exactly why the incoming phones weren't being answered. They explained that they had been instructed not to answer incoming calls until their outgoing calls were complete. With the paper mountain as it was, there was no realistic expectation of completion so the incoming lines were invariably ignored.

They were very aware that this wasn't right, but didn't feel they had a right to challenge management instructions. They explained their frustration that they were working normal office hours and that many of the people they were trying to ring were likely doing the same.

One said that she got quite excited when a human being actually answered the phone. She explained that in order to protect patient confidentiality, she was not allowed to leave answerphone messages, so was very conscious that somewhere in the region of 60-70% of her working time was adding no value. In her words she felt *'pointless and voiceless'*.

I asked the group whether there were a few simple changes that could be made to improve things. The solutions were obvious to everyone who had endured the working arrangements.

The next day we re-grouped to put our plan into action. The team was split into two, with half taking incoming calls, and half making outgoing calls to patients identified by their dates of birth as being more likely to be at home to receive day time calls. The groups rotated once every hour to ease monotony.

The paper mountain was removed to another location close by so that the team saw a manageable pile of letters to tackle during the single shift.
The team were asked to consider changing working hours to include hours when working patients were more likely to be at home.

All were keen to contribute to this as they were *'determined to shrink the paper mountain'*.

And finally – in response to a heart-wrenching plea for refreshment, a water cooler was installed in the corner of the cabin so the team could have chilled water on tap.

That weekend, a deep clean of the porta-cabin was arranged which drastically improved the working environment.

The positive impact of these changes was felt immediately, and two weeks later, the recorded percentage of aborted incoming calls reduced from 55% to 3%.
Having worked as a frazzled operational manager myself, it is important to acknowledge the luxury of seeing opportunities for improvement from the outside looking in.

I am absolutely sure that there have been times when I would have been one of the managers contributing to the *blame the absent party* manoeuvre. I can genuinely empathise with the tendency to keep things creaking along to avoid the disruption of change.

Resistance to change is a very well documented human reaction. As is resistance to doing something because you believe it is what someone else wants.

I guess my challenge to you is to see if you can resist the urge to resist.

If you are brave and genuinely believe that the inevitable difficulties and disruption will be worthwhile in the end, then go for it.

(Unless, of course, what is being suggested is genuinely bonkers. In which case you have my permission to refuse!)

Power struggles and resistance

This subject is worthy of a book of it's own. I may write one!

For the purposes of this guide I will merely scratch the surface.

I feel that I should disclose at this point, that I have a strong fascination with the relationship between clinicians and non-clinical managers.

My interest came from early observations of doctors and managers working together (or, in some cases, not working together), within clinical specialties.

You will remember that I had come from the outside world of work and knew nothing about the NHS, and that I had previously worked in jobs where every minute had a clear purpose towards delivering something tangible.

So, as an outsider looking in, I was struck by how little positive interaction there was between the expert professional staff providing clinical services to patients, and those responsible for making sure budgets balanced and targets were met.

And when the two 'sides' (I say sides because it often felt like sides), came together, I heard really odd conversations about managers *caring more about targets than people'* and doctors *'doing their own thing with no interest in the wider service'*.

I recently shared a very interesting 90 minutes with a clinical leader who I will call Dr X. As is often the case, a non-clinical manager had called me in to support this consultant to understand 'how to improve as a leader'.

As I approached the leader's office, I guessed that whilst I might be about to meet a clinical leader who could improve (as could we all!), I might also be about to meet a human being as keen to succeed as the manager but coming at the challenge from a different angle.

I was right.

The conversation went something like this.

Dr X: *I'm not entirely sure why I am meeting you.*

Me: *Well, my understanding is that I am at your disposal to support you with anything you might be finding challenging in your leadership role. Shall we start with things you find frustrating?*

Dr X: *How long have you got?*
(The ice is broken)

Dr X: *Do you know what gets to me more than anything else?*

Dr X went on to tell me about his regret at ever putting himself forward to be a clinical leader. He said he felt ill equipped to do the job. He talked about finding time to be a leader while he maintained a heavy clinical workload. He talked about non-clinical managers having so little understanding of the difficulties he faced. He talked about overhearing a colleague say that he had *'stopped being a decent bloke when he crossed the management line'*.

Not long afterwards, I had a conversation with another clinical leader who had a reputation (amongst the non-clinical managers) for being a very difficult person to deal with.

My work had previously bought me into close contact with him as he undertook a complex clinical research project. He worked silly hours of the day and night and was absolutely passionate about using the research to make a difference to patients' lives.

Yet, this was a man who simply refused to co-operate with anything suggested to him by anyone who was a manager (or in any way resembled one).

I spoke to him about why people might experience him as 'difficult' when, by all accounts he was an excellent doctor who was clearly hugely liked and respected by his patients.

We had a really good chat. He told me that he had nothing whatsoever against any one that he worked with. He told me that if he were to meet them in another part of his life, he would probably get on just fine with them.

He also told me that when he had dreamed of being a doctor, he had never imagined, for one minute, that there would be so much bureaucracy around the relatively straightforward process of meeting, treating and supporting patients. He said that he loved every minute he spent with his patients; he enjoyed projects that had clear outcomes, but that he hated every minute he was required to engage in leadership activities that he believed had no purpose.

He promised to try harder to be nice but added that it was really hard when he saw so many things going on around him that really had no point at all.

I think what I took away from these meetings, and from similar encounters from disgruntled (but otherwise reasonable) clinical leaders, is just how ill equipped they can feel to challenge their peers, and how intolerable the bureaucratic processes and systems around them can feel.

Now is not the time to bore you with the history of NHS management and the well-documented erosion of clinical autonomy since the 1980s. I do, however, believe that the mismatch between expected professional freedoms and reality of experience persist to this day.

For this reason, I personally find it really helpful to cut clinical leaders a little slack when facing active resistance. A bit of genuine listening to fears and frustrations can allow the door to open far enough to get a toe in.

Once you get to that stage, why not have a go at approaching a contentious subject from a less threatening perspective. I quite like this one.

'Imagine we didn't both think that this change/ idea/ initiative was ridiculous, might it be worth at least exploring the concept?'

If the idea is inherently a good one, this might set you off on a positive path where you can bring your mutual skills to the table. You may, of course, conclude that the suggestion from 'The Management' is not actually very helpful at all.

However, if you have challenged yourselves to look for the good, you will be far better equipped to objectively respond with a counter suggestion. The important thing is to discourage resistance for the sake of resistance, and to make sure you add genuine value with your alternative ideas.

There is nothing more pleasing to me than seeing a visible shift from resistance towards a positive solution. Or when cries of '**they** want us to do something' are replaced by 'why don't **we** try that'.

Self-awareness

A few years ago I had a quite dreadful weekend following a meeting at work that did not go well. The meeting was at 4pm on a Friday. I didn't sleep at-all on the Friday night. I spent the entire weekend thinking, thinking and thinking again about what had happened.

The story is still quite painful to recall, but in summary followed a request by a member of my team to meet with her staff. She said they had some concerns. She didn't elaborate further and the meeting was set for two days later.

As background to what followed, the meeting happened at a time when I was fighting to keep the team funded. External funding for their work was coming to an end. Money was very scarce across the organisation. Behind the scenes I was trying every possible route to keep the team in place. And, at the same time, I was facing growing pressure to use our limited budget in a different way.

As I walked into the room, hostility hit me like a juggernaut.

I was told, in no uncertain terms, that I didn't care. Frustration and concern hit me from all corners of the room. One member of the team crossed the line of acceptable behaviour with a personal attack that can only be described as vicious and vindictive.
It cut so deep that I still recoil when I recall the exact words he used.

I think what hurt most was that some of what was being said immediately resonated as understandable from staff fearing for their livelihoods. Their manager was in the room and I was disappointed to see her joining in with the assault as each member of the team gained courage from their colleagues.

I would like to believe that I stayed relatively calm though every part of me wanted to cry and to scream injustice. I know that my efforts not to break fuelled their perception of my cold heart even further.

Whilst I could go on, and provide the sordid details of the ordeal and its aftermath, it is enough to say that I learned a great deal from the encounter.

Once I'd got over the hurt and sense of injustice, I found myself reflecting on what had made the team so angry, and why their anger was so clearly directed at me, personally.

The fact was that the weeks leading up to this day had been extremely stressful, and everywhere I turned I was being told that there were too many pulls on budgets and that the team I had built was not essential to 'core business'.

So whilst I was struggling to be heard; sleeping very little, and trying to keep control of my emotions, my behaviour was being perceived as 'cold and uncaring' by a team of staff who were fearful of losing their jobs.

The fact was, they had no idea what was going on behind the scenes to try and save the service. I had somehow overlooked the fact that sharing this might have been helpful to them.

In the absence of facts from me, they had been speculating, and building a growing picture of me as an insensitive manager who was doing absolutely nothing to support their plight.

In the exercise that follows I am asking you to reflect on your own behaviour at work when things have been particularly stressful.

I believe that reflecting on how others might perceive you in these situations can be really helpful for you, and for those around you.

So as you take a deep breath and lay yourself bare, think about some times at work when (normally reasonable) people have been critical of you, or when you knew deep down that your own behaviour got in the way of doing the right thing.

Think about whether you might recognise your own behaviour in any of the statements below

Be kind to yourself when doing this exercise. It's about learning to recognise your tendencies and learn from them. It's not about beating yourself up for being human.

When you've finished, check below to see what might have been driving your inner voices.

THE SELF-AWARENESS EXERCISE

1. Why would I put myself through that? It's going to disrupt things and make people annoyed.

2. I'm pretty sure there are other people better equipped to deal with this than me.

3. I don't agree with this but I'm going to keep quiet in case I look stupid.

4. I'll let her/him be the one to tell her/him. That way I don't have to face the fallout.

5. I know it's the right thing to do, but if they go for that it will impact me personally.

6. I know I'm right but I'm getting bored arguing the point so I will let it go.

7. I know I'm rubbish so I'm not going to put myself forward.

8. I know better than anyone in this room so I'll say yes but I'm not going to do it.

9. I get what I'm being asked to do, but if I keep doing it my way it will be a lot easier for me.

10. I know this isn't of much benefit any more but I enjoy it so we'll carry on.

11. I don't know why I can't just tell people what's happening rather than ask them what they think.

12. I don't think people have the same moral code as I do.

13. Everyone is praising the team but I led it, at the end of the day so a bit of singling out would be good.

14. I don't care who wants it done that way, its fine the way it is.

15. I really wish I could just get on with this on my own rather than involve other people.

16. I will talk about other things and hope no one wants an answer on that one.

Now let's consider what might have been driving those thoughts.

If you recognised 1, 2, 4 and/or 16, perhaps your inner voice was one of self-preservation?

If you recognised 3, 7 and/or 9, perhaps your inner voice was one of self-consciousness or self-doubt?

If you recognised 5, 8, and/or 14, perhaps your inner voice was one of self-interest?

If you recognise 6,11 and/or 13, perhaps your inner voice was one of self-importance or plain arrogance (!)?

If you recognised 10, perhaps your inner voice was one of self-indulgence?

If you recognised 12, perhaps your inner voice was one of self-righteousness?

If you recognised 15, perhaps your inner voice was one of self-sufficiency?

These are by no means all of the 'self' subjects that might come in to play.

The important thing is that awareness of your personal needs, fears and desires can help you understand the negative reactions that they trigger – and to work on them.

Allowable weaknesses?

I often come across management and leadership behaviour that other people tell me is a problem. For example:

Please can you talk to Samantha. She is upsetting people by the way she talks to them.

Please can you observe Dr Costello He's great in a lot of ways but anything that touches on certain subjects sets him off into a sulk.

We are really struggling to understand Martyn. He's great 1:1 but very quiet in meetings.

When I meet Samantha, Dr Costello or Martyn, we usually have a good chat, and the reasons for their behaviours come to the surface, or, at least, a little closer to it. At best the issue is resolved with the help of a good conversation. More likely, the conversation goes some way towards exposing the root cause; supporting reflection and improved self-awareness.

This is not a psychology textbook, so suffice to say that behaviours perceived by others as an issue will likely have their roots in a myriad of causes. - Personality, culture, experience, bias, assumption, to name but a few.

Most healthcare leaders I meet can identify at least one colleague whose behaviour drives them potty. It is usually more than one!

I once met a manager from a back-office corporate function who we will call Linda. One of the first things I learned about Linda was that she had a propensity for sending very long emails. Not necessarily a crime in its own right, but it was the content that struck me.

In response to even simple requests for information you pretty much knew that the reply would include numerous seemingly friendly statements each with a little sting attached.

For example:

It is so lovely to hear from you. I am very happy to provide this information. Obviously, I am curious about why you would want it as I have already provided it many times before but that is fine.

Or

I am sure you will know from your vast experience that these things aren't easy, so if you have any tips for me about how you have achieved what no one else seems able to, I'd be very happy to meet you for coffee and talk about them.

Or

I am so pleased (my boss) has called you in to do something he has already asked me to do. Not sure why to be honest but we always enjoy having you around.

In person, the passive aggressive tone continued:

It's so lovely to see you. Why are you getting involved in our work again did you say?

It's great that you want to do things so quickly. I guess it's easy for you because this is the only thing you're doing.

Thank you so much for coming in today especially to see us. You really didn't need to.

Linda genuinely believed herself to be extremely busy. Her diary was filled with meetings, and with meetings about meetings. Linda very rarely challenged herself to see things from different perspectives. Sadly, her managers had long since abandoned their efforts to challenge her.

When you recognise passive aggressive behaviour in colleagues, at any level, I strongly advise you to be willing and courageous and to tackle it gently but directly. Skilfully handled, you may expose a root cause that can be addressed or at least deliver a clear message that behaviour that makes the workplace unpleasant for others is not something that can be entertained in any circumstances.

My next example is an exposé of my own behaviour. I know I will feel uncomfortable sharing it even though it happened many years ago. I will admit that the incident is at the back of my mind most of the time, and can leap to the fore when I observe similar behaviour in others.

I am a lot older and, (I'd like to believe), a little bit wiser now, but as a young manager learning my trade I know I was guilty of less than ideal behaviour on numerous occasions.

In particular, I have a natural tendency to expect ludicrously high standards of work from myself and from everyone I work with. For many reasons (some of which I guess might be better exposed through therapy!), I have always been driven to complete every working task to the very best of my ability. Not from the perspective of ego or status, I might add, but because in the early days of my career, I derived much of my self worth and self respect from the quality of work I delivered.

On one occasion, a long time before I joined healthcare, I was managing a team who were responsible for delivering a high profile project on budget and on time. The project was absolutely time critical, as was the need for extremely careful budget management. It was a >£1million project where literally every penny mattered.

The project was a creative one, and I was working with some extremely talented people who, by their nature, were less inclined to focus on detail, and more on creating a fantastic product.

As the project progressed, pressure to deliver on time and within budget was immense. The reputation of the company would stand or fall on delivery. I took this pressure home. I lived it, breathed it and slept with it (or, more frequently didn't sleep).

And it took its toll.

I became more and more stressed and more and more dissatisfied with colleagues who seemed disinterested in the things I believed to be important.

Everything came to a head when I walked into the project office one morning following a call from a supplier. The supplier's bill had not been paid despite being sent in to the office 6 weeks earlier.

As I approached the office I heard the sound of creative banter. I would not ordinarily have a problem with this and, at my best, I would be right in there amongst it. But on this particular day, the banter took on what I perceived to be a disregard for urgency.

One of my colleagues was really untidy, and on her desk I spotted a very big pile of papers with some invoices on top.

This particular colleague hadn't yet arrived at work. I asked where she was and was told she was coming in late. This would not ordinarily have been problem to me, as this team always worked hours well over and above the call of duty.

And then it happened.

The actions I took put in place a chain of events that was to prove more damaging than I could ever imagine, and which, to this day, sends cold shivers down my spine.

I found myself grabbing at the pile of papers and frantically searching through them to find the unpaid invoice. I found it towards the bottom of the pile.

Finding it there triggered panic that if this could happen, I clearly did not have sufficient grip and control on the project.

Fighting back tears, I took the pile of papers to my office and spurting out to colleagues that I wanted to see the owner of the pile as soon as she arrived at work.

By the time my colleague sought me out, I had calmed down. I tried my best to explain to her why I had reacted as I did. I clumsily tried to reaffirm the importance of dealing with paperwork, not stacking it up. But the damage was done.

We were all quite young, we were all immature and insecure and I was immediately cast in the role of volatile, unfair, untrusting manager.

As I recoil from the memory with the benefit of many years of hindsight, I know exactly what was driving my behaviour.

I'm not excusing it in any way but at least now can reconcile that it came from my very deep-rooted fear of getting things wrong and there being consequences.

Over time, you may have come to some sort of conclusion about why people you work with behave as they do. You may be right. You may be wrong. My challenge is for you to resist the urge to make an early judgement and to question whether what is being observed might possibly be symptomatic of circumstances, or something that can be positively addressed. Any insight you gain into possible or probable cause of the behaviour you're seeing can be used to initiate a careful conversation.

Remember that challenge of behaviour is a tricky and sensitive area, but one that the best leaders bravely face head on.

My advice is to proceed with caution and sensitivity using skill, will and plenty of courage.

Adding real value

For managers and leaders spending every day fire fighting to keep afloat (excuse me muddling the elements!), it can be extremely difficult to stand back and ask the question:

'Hold on. Am I actually adding value here?'

If you make a conscious effort to ask yourself that question a few times a day, or even once, at the end of each day, it might be wise to prepare yourself for an unexpected answer. You may, for example, find that you have spent the day expending massive effort in simply stopping anything bad from happening. Keeping the service running when a critical person is away, perhaps. Or keeping a couple of warring colleagues from letting their issues spill out and cause damage to others. Or discovering a quick work around to a failing system or process.

On days like this, you can give yourself a gentle pat on the back for succeeding in damage limitation. The enhanced value you can bring is to apply skill will and courage to resolving the underlying issues.

The days when the pat on your back can be considerably harder is when you reflect on instances where you stepped way out of your comfort zone to do the right thing in spite of the odds.

Then there will be the days when you ask yourself the question and you have to conclude that you added little value, other than warming your chair, or worse, behaving in a way that got in the way of progress.

Those times when you were perhaps a little disrespectful towards colleagues; thought more of *self* than of the greater good; let your ego do the talking, or disregarded all views expect your own. There was once a manager. We will call her Anna.

She was extremely professional in her appearance. She came to work every day, come rain or shine. She arrived promptly at 8am. So far, so good, you may be thinking.

Anna had been a manager for a long time. She was always keen to let people know how close to the top of her profession she had risen, and how she had chosen, in more recent years, to work in a position that was actually a little beneath her ability.

I was involved in a working project that involved Anna and her team. She was very concerned about the idea of me meeting members of her team without her being present. She had the air of someone completely in control of her life and keen to control everything around her at work.

Anna resided over a team of administrative staff. Her role was one that maintained an oversight over administration. Her job title also suggested that she was the more appropriate go-to person for value adding professional activities. In our first meeting, she proceeded to criticise everyone and everything around her. She told me how good she was at what she does – adding that she couldn't really do any of the things she is so good at because of things that get in the way. She told me how awful the senior managers were. She speculated as to their qualifications and suitable experience for office.

I dared to suggest that there might possibly be some opportunities to improve working processes within her area of administration. She told me all the reasons why my ideas wouldn't work. She also told me many reasons why her organisation was unique and why things that might have worked elsewhere wouldn't work in her service.

She showed me her diary. It was full of meetings that she attended across the week. How helpful are those in supporting you to drive progress? I asked. They are all pointless she replied.

This is a lady who will likely continue in this vein for a few more years yet.

I sometimes describe encounters like this as times when I find people who have somehow *blended into the walls* of the healthcare institutions they work in. There is no part of me that believes it is OK to accept this as any kind of norm.

Do you know an Anna or two where you work? Would you overlook this behaviour in yourself or others?

I was once asked to observe a hospital Board in action and to provide unfiltered feedback of my observations. The Board was preparing for an external assessment that would specifically measure effectiveness of both the Board as a whole, and of each person around the Board table.

If you are familiar with Board structures, you will know that these comprise Executive and Non-Executive Board members. Each of the Executives has accountabilities relating to specific subject areas alongside a level of shared responsibility for organisational effectiveness.

In UK healthcare, the Non-Executive Directors hold the Executives to account via appropriate challenge and scrutiny, and also play their part in sharing responsibility for success. Or so they should.

To gather the necessary information for my feedback, I attended three meetings in quick succession. The first was a full public Board meeting. The second was the confidential Board session that routinely follows each public meeting. The third was the weekly Executive Management meeting held the day after the Board.

The first meeting started well and I observed some great value adding exchanges between members of the Board. Next came a great presentation from the Director of Nursing and two members of her team.

It went downhill from there.

One of the Non-Executive Directors looked out from over his glasses and drew members of the Board to the attention of a typing error on page 17 of an Appendix. Here we go, I thought. Everyone scrambled through the committee papers.

From the sidelines I looked on in eager anticipation.

Would the error be a critical one?

Had someone inadvertently added a nought to the critical finance figures, or something that materially changed the content in a worrying way?

No. It was a misplaced apostrophe.

It honestly was.

Now you may believe this to be insignificant but here's how the situation escalated.

The Executive Directors were clearly rattled. The mood of the meeting changed, and as each Director stood to deliver their reports there was a palpable air of defence. As questions were asked, the directors seemed flummoxed. They fluffed their lines. This, in turn gave fuel to Mr Apostrophe who appeared to relish their fears and ignite them further.

Fast forward to the Executive meeting the next day and a good hour of the bulging business agenda was taken up in an ill mannered exchange of views about the Board meeting the previous day.

Exec 1: *But you know what's he's like. Why didn't you check the report better?*

Exec 2: *Give me a break. He was going to find something in one of the papers.*

Exec 3: *OK everyone. Let's talk about the actions from yesterday.*

Exec 4: *No. We need to talk about how (Mr Apostrophe) makes us all feel.*

Exec 5: *Yes we need to do that.*

Cue a fairly meaningless discussion with much disagreement and eye rolling. Noticeably, no one suggested that perhaps it would be helpful to have a proper discussion with Mr Apostrophe, or the fact that their collective inability to handle him was significantly reducing the effectiveness of the Board.

You may or may not sit around the Board table in your own organisation. You may have visited the Board and observed the members in action. Or you may never have experienced your Board first hand.

Whatever your role in relation to the Board, I have a challenge for you.

Find a way to attend your Board in the guise of an outsider looking in. Suspend any preconception or assumption, if you can, and objectively assess what you see from the perspective of *added-value.* You may see nothing but cohesive, value adding excellence from start to finish. Or not.

Be really honest in your observations then challenge yourself to do something with them. Feedback like this takes a very healthy dose of courage!

Blindly following the leader

I have come across a few managers and leaders who make the mistake of believing they are always right.

Of these, the most arrogant also believe that there is little value in listening to different points of view, as it merely wastes time. They are invariably wrong.

More worrying than this, is when I watch how these managers operate and see people around them going along with everything they say without so much as a *'Are you sure that's the only way?'*

I worked in an organisation that was good but could have been even better.

The most senior leader was supremely articulate, clever and committed to the cause. She also had extremely fixed ideas about people she liked and those she didn't.

Early on, I saw her taking a particular dislike to two people I believed to have great potential as leaders.

I came to realise that her decision to keep people within her favoured pool was directly related to her ability to mould them to her likeness, and to blindly agree with her.

Over time, her close circle became so blinded by her influence, that I witnessed intelligent, decent people who had previously challenged injustice and known their own minds, speaking extremely disrespectfully about anyone not considered worthy of a place within the clique.

Whilst I don't want to fill this guide with management jargon, a technical term that came to mind in this particular situation was that I was witnessing *groupthink*. This term relates to a situation where the need and desire for conforming to a particular view, or course of action, overrides the desire and ability to challenge.

I have absolutely no doubt that individuals surrounding this leader fell victim to this and, as a result, missed some pretty important opportunities to become great.

This particular leader was particularly complex, but she certainly isn't the only one I've met that has played more the role of pied piper than effective, inclusive leader.

My challenge here is for you to reflect on whether you might possibly be a leader that always believes you're right? Or are you one that takes people with you for the wrong reasons? Or might you possibly be tempted to blindly follow to be one of the favoured few?

Beyond average

You may recall that earlier in this guide I referred to

the senior leader who, by his own admission, was *aspiring to be average.* I was perturbed by his view, but as I got to know the system better, I must admit that I understood a little of what he was saying.

With challenges round every corner, and relentless pressure to do more, with less, you may well find yourself choosing which battles should be fought. You may also find relative peace and comfort in keeping your head slightly beneath the parapet to avoid too much scrutiny.

This may sound harsh; so let me elaborate with an example of average (at best) in action. In my work, I have the luxury of observing many healthcare leaders at work. I know that it is far easier to be objective as an outsider looking in. I also know that leaders can become so embroiled in the politics and complexities of their organisations, that they may not spot a growing tendency to keep heads down.

I spent some time working in a healthcare organisation that is widely recognised for its ground breaking clinical work. My work bought me into close contact with the hospital's Executive Management Team. The work I was bought in to do was absolutely achievable, but I quickly realised that there was a fundamental underlying issue that would inevitably rear its head on my departure if the root causes weren't addressed.

Not one to shy away from a tricky discussion, I took the bull by the horns and secured a slot on the weekly Executive meeting agenda. My slot in that initial session went something like this.

Thank you very much for giving me the opportunity to meet with you today. I'm not sure how much each of you knows about why I've come here, so I thought it would be helpful to summarise and also to let you know some of the things I've picked up straight away which might help us succeed. For me, it's really important that I don't just come in and do something and walk away, but also that what we achieve, together, is sustained.

Ice broken, I took a deep breath and launched into my observations, and the reasons why I could make quick changes but that they would only be lasting with their help and commitment.

There was some interesting looks around the table which I interpreted, in one case, to a *'who does she think she is?'* reaction, and, in another, to discomfort that the issues were familiar. I sensed that that person knew what needed to be done but perhaps had not had the skill, will or courage to take action herself.

I paused for breath and invited comment and the excuses came thick and fast.

'With all due respect', said the one who had previously rolled his eyes at my suggestion that we might share some responsibility for improvement.

He repeated *'With all due respect, isn't this what we've bought you in to do. I'm not sure what it's got to do with us'.*

His colleague chipped in. *'No. To be fair, I understand that, as leaders we need to be involved. Maybe you could write us a monthly report while you're here'.*

Another colleague joined in. *'Thinking about it a bit more, the people we bring in to do things like this aren't usually that good. Its looks like they've done something but it never seems to last. Sorry, but what makes you different?'*

Doing my best to bite my tongue without drawing blood, I said that I was not actually asking for much

103

over and above two commitments from the Executive team.

The first was that they were prepared to say – out loud – that they believed the change we were looking to introduce was the right thing to do.

The second was that when I had gone, and people around them were having a wobble at keeping things going, that they would hold their nerve and keep steering in the right direction.

What happened next stopped me in my tracks.

Everyone round the table burst into spontaneous laughter. The first words I heard emerge from the mirth were

'Yes. We never do that; we're rubbish at that'.

This was no laughing matter and I think I may just have stopped my mouth dropping fully open at this point.

My realisation that this team was completely blind to both their collective corporate accountability and to their critical role in challenging the status quo shocks me to this day.

Finding support

In your day-to-day role as a healthcare leader, people doubtless come at you from all angles expecting you to be the font of all knowledge.

People around you can be very quick to judge any perceived gaps in your knowledge, behaviour that is less than perfect or views that may be contrary to their own.

However resilient and self sufficient you may think you are, it is always good to know that there is a safe place to go for a quick scream and download. I quite specifically say a 'quick' scream and download as I have seen colleagues falling into a habit of perpetual download. Watch out for signs of yourself and others falling into the trap of the one-hour work to one-hour despair ratio. It is never healthy.

Support networks can come from unlikely sources, and my advice is always to look out for a friendly ear that understands your pain. Search out those that lead you away from the path of over-indulgence, but who get what you're saying, and are able to offer a positive perspective.

Personally, I tend to seek out colleagues who understand that the system is bonkers but remains determined to make a difference – Or can convince me that whilst individuals can sometimes be mad / bad / odd / difficult / infuriating, it doesn't (always) mean those people are beyond help and support.

Those, I find, are the very best supporters.

As a leader, you have to remember that there are times when despite drawing on you deepest reserves of skill, will and courage, you might find yourself out of your depth and in need of support from other angles.

There is absolutely no shame in this and a deep breath in followed by exhalation of the words *'I have absolutely no idea how to tackle this, can you help?'* can save many hours, day and nights of worry and stress.

Sadly, I have encountered many a manager reluctant to ask for help, support or advice. Reasons for the resistance vary a lot. From *'my senior manager would expect me to know that'* to *'I need to deal with this one on my own'* to '*It's my fault we're in this position'*.

It wasn't that many years ago when I woke up one day and realised it was OK not to know everything that I might possibly encounter at work. It was such a revelation. I do also know that pride; stupidity, fear and many other factors can get in the way of the words *'I need your help'.*

Nowadays, I thoroughly enjoy supporting those who use the *'my manager would expect me to know that'* line.

'Well if that's the case', I say, *'your manager obviously knows the answer so might be able to share it with you…. Go on…. Ask them'….*

The managers who do know the answer tend to be only too willing to share their superior knowledge. If they are a little smug whilst sharing their wisdom, it is absolutely fine. You have the answer you need.

The managers who don't know the answer might get a little defensive. But you can rest assured that if they're decent they will admit it and bowl in to help you find out.

If you are ever in doubt or out of your depth, be courageous and ask.

Meetings

I've given the subject of meetings a heading of its own because, prior to healthcare, I never worked anywhere else where so many diaries are jam-packed with so many meetings. To be clear, I can think of plenty of jobs where managers might appropriately spend a lot of time in the presence of other people.

What I really mean is that I had never seen diaries crammed with so many meetings that have so little to do with actually getting things done.

Before your hackles rise at any suggestion that I might be questioning the way you spend your time, I feel I need to explain this a little bit more.

Be honest now. Have you ever sat in a work meeting and wondered what you were doing there? What value the meeting was adding? Whether your time might be better spent getting on with the job in hand?

Not long into my healthcare service, I attended a committee meeting where the first hour of the two hour meeting was spend reviewing progress on the actions arising from the previous meeting.

As each subject was raised, the person responsible for updating drew attention to a paper that they had written to provide evidence of progress. All these papers were extremely comprehensive.

Each author then asked if members of the Committee had had the opportunity to read the paper. Most said no as it had only been circulated 24 hours before the meeting. *'No matter'*, said each author, *'I will take you through the key points now'*. As each author stepped forward to present, I was struck by the defensive nature of each presentation.

'So, as you will see from the progress graph, we haven't made the progress we had hoped to'

'As you will see from the figures, what we presented last month was overly optimistic'

'This paper explains the progress we will be taking to undertake the actions next month that you asked us to undertake last month'.

More shocking than my sense of things not progressing, was the response from the Chair thanking the presenters for their *'extremely helpful updates'*. To me, this suggested that reporting on a lack of progress was something quite normal and acceptable to the organisation. In all of my work before joining healthcare, the concept of a meeting that did nothing other than reporting on no-progress would have been inconceivable.

Conversely, I had the privilege to attend a number of clinically focused meetings in my early days – Multidisciplinary meetings where doctors discuss the best course of action for their most complexly unwell patients. These meetings were focussed on agreeing exactly what to do, and making sure it happened.

The longer I spent amongst managers and clinical leaders the more I realised that whilst some meetings are essential for complex decision making, or as part of formal governance or communication arrangements, many fail to deliver anything concrete, or serve a purpose that could be equally well served over a quick coffee catch-up, a much swifter face to face encounter, or a different mode of information sharing.

In almost every organisation I support these days, there will be some sort of initiative in place to reduce the length of meetings, reduce the number of meetings, have better focus in meetings, make meeting papers shorter and smarter... You get the picture.

Yet despite this, a glance at managers' calendars reveals endless round of operations' meetings, performance meetings, quality meetings, improvement meetings, project meetings, safety meetings, risk meetings, innovation meetings, value meetings. Again, you get the picture.

Recognising that a culture of over-meeting & under-doing still prevails in some quarters, my challenge to you is to join your more courageous colleagues in proffering alternative positive solutions.
Bear in mind that a simple refusal to attend a meeting that someone else thinks is absolutely essential is unlikely to go down well.

Perhaps, reflect on what the meetings is actually trying to achieve, and find a way to frame an alternative solution to achieving the same end without so much staring and sparring across a meeting table.

Pause for reflection

CHAPTER 4
FROM SURVIVING TO THRIVING

So far, we've talked a lot about survival

Now I will challenge you to reflect on the extent to which you are going beyond skin-of-your-teeth survival, to thriving personally and professionally in the complex and illogical world that we call healthcare.

From personal experience, I strongly believe that one of the ways to leap from surviving to thriving comes from a realisation that the system is a long way from perfect, but that some fairly hefty mountains can be moved by taking a deep breath; catching a fair wind, and venturing forth with a healthy dose of skill, will and courage.

It also helps to conclude that a vast majority of people you work with are likely to be decent and reasonable human beings. They may be driven by their own needs and desires, and you might not always see them at their best, but, deep down most of them will be as committed as you are to doing what's right for patients.

Of course, there will be one or two (possibly more) who will test your resolve; make you doubt yourself, or make you want to run for the hills.

You'll need to decide for yourself how to handle these people and which battles to fight.

My only plea is that you do your upmost to stick to your guns and your instinct. Dig in your heels if you need to. Focus on doing what's right, and don't let anyone dent your confidence or take up negative space in your head.

Oh. And if you realise that the job you're doing, or the place you're doing it in, just aren't for you, don't be scared to grab the bull by the proverbial horns and find another place to apply your talents.

Bravery, resilience and tenacity can shift entrenched attitudes and positions; win hearts and minds; bring ideas to life, and unite folks in the belief that change can be for the good.

I'm not going to promise this will be easy.

The leap from surviving to thriving demands bucket loads of positive energy; supporting and encouraging those who find change difficult, and tirelessly driving progress, despite the system and despite the detractors.

A trivial story that has stuck in my mind relates to a manager who we will call Judith.

I was working alongside a clinical team in a hospital to help identify ways we could improve a process. We had come up with some solutions that we had to present to a committee in the form of a report.

I drafted the report and circulated it to Judith and the five other managers involved. I received some helpful comments in return, but nothing from Judith. I prompted her twice.

I received a short sharp email in response.

"I have considered the report you have written and would advise you that the font you have used isn't the one we usually use here".

I thanked her for her reply and asked if she had anything she wanted to add about the content.

No reply.

Judith had been an NHS manager for a long time. So I guess we could call her a survivor. But I couldn't help wondering whether she'd once aspired for more, and whether she would be altogether happier if she believed thriving to be an option.

I mentioned earlier the idea of *blending into the walls* of an organisation and I believe we have all come across colleagues whose behaviour or *'funny little ways'* is excused as in inevitable by product of working for a large organisation.

I struggle with the idea that any manager or leader would get up in the morning content with the idea of spending their day protecting themselves from the notion of managing or leading! Sadly, though, I have come across quite a few Judiths who have been all but forgotten and left to their own devices.

Personally, I believe there is absolutely no shame in concluding that managing or leading isn't for you, and that your organisation would get the best from you in a role that allows you to play to different strengths.

For example, I have worked with many clinicians keen to pursue leadership roles who struggle with the loss of clinical workload; who quickly lose the will to battle systems or who genuinely struggle with the idea of challenging their colleagues.

For some of these leaders, a return to clinical practice is inevitable. For others, there is nothing more satisfying than watching them grow through challenges; applying increasing skill, will and courage to triumph and thrive against the odds.

In the same way as I believe there is no shame in admitting defeat in the personal battle between clinical practice and leadership, I also have no problem with the idea that an individual's skills, willingness and courage may not be suited to a particular organisation.

In my work I have had the privilege to dip in and out of a large number of healthcare organisations and I have yet to come across one that doesn't have quirks and characters in need of support! In a vast majority of cases, I see decent people and good intentions all around me.

However, in all of the organisations, I make a point of asking myself the question
'If I were to consider working in a permanent role, would I thrive as a manager / leader here?'

117

This may seem like an odd question for me to ask myself.

I urge you to ask yourself the same question of the organisation you are currently working in.

I also urge you to expand your questioning as follows:

- *Appreciating that we're all under pressure, do the people around me want the same things for the patients as I do?*

- *If I were feeling overwhelmed would I have a safe outlet here for sharing my worries?*

- *Am I able to forgive odd behaviour in colleagues as 'allowable weaknesses'?*

- *Appreciating we all have good and bad days, do I usually get out of bed reasonably content to be venturing into work?*

- *Am I comfortable that the interests of the patients and the organisation over and above self-interest motivate my colleagues?*

I firmly believe that whilst a career in healthcare management or leadership is not for the fainthearted, it should also be one where there is a high level of support and satisfaction.

So, in the days that feel like 2 steps forward and one and a half steps backwards, the half step forward can be celebrated with like-minded colleagues. Likewise, the one and a half steps backwards can be accepted as a given with some peer-empathy and a good dose of humour (where appropriate!)

Conversely, if the constant forward and backward steps feel lonely; with no-one around to either celebrate of commiserate, or worst still, with folks around you looking to find fault, then it would be entirely justifiable to question whether your skill, will and courage might be better applied elsewhere.

Life is short and work is a big part of it. Please don't waste it flogging dead horses.

On a more positive note, I've been around and about long enough to learn that the healthcare leaders who are brave, and who strive, relentlessly, not to blend into the walls, are amongst the most inspired and inspiring people I could ever hope to meet.

You work exceptionally hard in an environment pressured from every single angle. You owe it to yourself to demand a work place that allows and encourages you to be the best you can be.

Pause for reflection

CHAPTER 5
THE WORKBOOK

This is the part of the book where I encourage you to find some quiet time, boil the kettle (or pour yourself a refreshing glass of something), and prepare to be challenged a little bit more.

The exercises that follow will test your skill, will and courage as far as you let them.

THE LEADERSHIP 'INCOMPETENCY' FRAMEWORK

This exercise is an irreverent nod to the numerous Leadership Development programmes I have attended over the years and a light-hearted way to explore a very serious subject.

I am making light of this to expose a very sensitive subject, and it's really important to remember that a lot of the behaviour you exhibit and observe at work may not be representative of people at their best or most comfortable.

Every day everyone brings to work a unique and complicated mix of skills, needs, fears, biases, interests, assumptions and expectations. Over time, the way you behave in the workplace becomes established and expected by your colleagues.

Holding a mirror up to yourself and others is a scary thing to do, but a brilliant way to take stock and make some changes if necessary.

Listed below are some less than helpful leadership behaviours I have genuinely witnessed over the past few years.

My challenge to you is to consider which of these traits you might personally have exhibited on your bad days, and/or which you may have seen in others.

- *When I arrive at work, I leave all logical thought processes at the door*

- *The multiple demands on my time leave me constantly stressed but I don't do anything about it*

- *I'm happy to sit through meetings that I know add no value*

- *The sound of an email pinging into the box fills me with dread so I leave it unopened*

- *I take my work home in my bag and in my head*

- *If someone else isn't prepared to do something, I don't see why I should*
- *If I need to do something difficult I won't do it until I'm chased*

- *If someone tells me something can't be done I will happily believe them*

- *If something's running OK, but not great, its best to leave it be*

- *If something isn't part of my job, you won't find me doing it*

- *I allow myself to get overwhelmed rather than ask for help*

- *I can't say no to anything asked of me*

- *When senior managers say jump, I say 'how high', even if I don't agree*

- *Even if I know something's right, I won't do it if its going to cause waves*

- *I can't fight the illogicality of it all. It is what it is.*

The Incompetency Framework is an exercise for reflection, not judgement. However, if you recognise more that a few of these traits on a regular basis, it may be time to have a good old chat with yourself.

ACTION AVOIDANCE BINGO

I'm pretty sure you'll be familiar with the various versions of Management Bingo kicking around.

The ones that talk about *getting your ducks in a row, on a burning platform while a giant ant is nipping at your ankles* (OK, I think I may have just made that last bit up).

As a tool for reflection, this game is a wee bit more serious than it may first appear.

I call it Action Avoidance Bingo.

The game is played over a period of 1-2 weeks.

All you need to do is make a note each time you hear yourself (or, if you prefer, one of your colleagues) utter one of the avoidance phrases.

When you have got to five have a think about whether the excuses were justifiable or whether they could possibly be masking an issue with skill, will or courage.

- *I'd love to but we won't be allowed*

- *It won't be yet because my diary's crazy*

- *We've tried that already*

- *I'll need to ask (next manager up)*

- *Good idea. Perhaps we could do it next year*

- *I don't think we can't trust the data*

- *I'll get my PA to arrange a meeting via your PA*

- *You'll need to ask (someone else)*

- *We should probably wait for the outcome of the review*

- *It won't get discussed this month, the agenda is full*

- *I thought we'd agreed someone else was dealing with that*

- *Can we talk about it once the holiday period is over*

- *That might work elsewhere but not around here*

- *It might be worth doing another review before we finally decide*

- *Why don't you set up another meeting so we can discuss it some more*

- *Yes, I do remember talking about it. It must have gone off my radar*

A 'BUT' FREE DAY

I recently spent some time working with a very inspirational leader who had banned the word 'but' from his business.

Working with him, I managed to ban it from my workday vocabulary (and pretty much from my home life too).

The habit stuck and although I am conscious I have used some 'buts' in this book, you can be assured each one had undergone scrutiny in the context of potential negative connotation!

Avoiding the use of 'but' when speaking, forces you to look for the positives in what you're hearing and to acknowledge them before proffering a positive idea on top.

Have a go at a 'but' free day and reflect on the impact.

REFRAMING THE ISSUE

You may have come across coaching techniques where you are encouraged to shift your perspective.

For example, you might be asked something like

'Imagine you could answer the question you are struggling to answer, what might your answer be?

or

'What might the cleverest person you know do in this situation?'

This tried and tested technique for re-framing a challenge can be extremely powerful in many different circumstances, both personal and professional.

Have a go at using this with something that you're finding really tricky to sort.

IT'S REALLY NOT PERSONAL

I have recently had the pleasure of supporting a lovely lady who was struggling with her self-confidence.

We'd got to the point where she was pretty sure she knew what had triggered her difficulties and she was showing a great determination to get back to her brightest and best.

So having established the strength of her commitment, I asked her if she thought she might be able to shift her perspective.

I asked her to do something she might find very odd.

I asked her to imagine that the person who had dented her confidence may not actually have meant to do so, but had, perhaps, acted clumsily as a result of her own lack of confidence, or another weakness in herself.

My coachee looked at me quizzically. We ended the session on that point of reflection.

The following day, I received one of those wonderful 'OMG' phone calls.

'I had to ring you. I thought about it and suddenly got it. I took what xxx said completely the wrong way. I watched her yesterday. She's really struggling with understanding some of her work and she's really stressed. It wasn't about me atall. I need to help her, don't I?'

In this challenge I'm asking you pick an upcoming working day and try to consciously react to other people's behaviour from a different perspective. Specifically, if you encounter anything negative from other people, tell yourself it's not personal. Decide that the negative behaviour is about the other person's situation rather than yours, and have a think about what the root cause may be.

I can't promise that you won't encounter behaviour that is just plain wrong, at times, but experience has told me that 9 out of 10 times, a shift in perspective can stop negativity in its tracks.

MINDING YOUR OWN BUSINESS

A few years ago, I worked with two clinical therapy teams whose managers had asked them to consider the possibility of working more closely together as most of their patients needed support from both professions. In particular, they had been asked to consider if it would be appropriate for their non-qualified assistants to learn and use skills related to both professions.

Their first response was quite defensive.

Working together in the way being suggested would undermine the individual professions, I was told. *This is a way for the hospital to employ less of us* one of the managers said.

So we approached the challenge from another angle.

I arranged a facilitated session for the two managers and a group of five of their staff from each profession.

In a relaxed environment away from the department, I asked them to imagine that they were running their own professional services' company, and that they were pitching to provide clinical services, across both of their professions to the hospital where they currently work.

By setting the challenge, hypothetically, from a different perspective, the managers and their staff immediately became more creative. They started to talk about how to do things most effectively and efficiently without undermining each other's expertise. When the conversation turned to support services, one of the staff suggested that they could *train up assistants to do different tasks to support the qualified clinicians from both professions.*

As is often the case, resistance gave way to a solution focus and individuals were assigned ownership of the project to make it happen.

So, consider a situation where you have resisted an initiative proposed by a senior manager. Ideally choose one you knew to be sensible, but for some reason you really didn't want to deal with it. Now imagine that you and the manager making the suggestion are actually partners in your own company, and that your income and reputation depends on making wise decisions.

How might you have reacted to the initiative in those circumstances?

WHAT'S THE POINT?

I recently had the pleasure of spending a day with a group of clinical managers whose own managers had signed them up to attend a day studying 'basic project management'. My brief was to support the managers with understanding the importance of finishing the numerous 'pieces of work' that land on their desks. So not really project management at all but I knew what they meant.

I decided to devote the first 45 minutes to giving the managers the opportunity to explain to me what they believed to be the issue.

Their concerns did not surprise me one bit.

'Often when we're given a piece-of-work its similar to a piece-of-work we've been given before which didn't really go anywhere. Its probably because when we receive pieces-of-work they have usually come about because someone from outside wants us to do something and we know it won't necessarily work but we have to do it anyway so we can tell the people that monitor us that we are doing it. And then something else comes along that isn't quite the same so we stop one piece of work and start another piece of work. And usually we have about 5 different

pieces of work going on and we're not quite sure why we're doing any of them. '

I decided that the session would be more valuably spent supporting the participants to challenge their tendency to accept *pieces of work* that they considered meaningless!

In this exercise, I challenge you to review everything in your current workload that falls into the category of *'a piece of work'* and to ask yourself, for each of these subjects, what is the point?

It could be that they are all clear, time bound, value adding projects - or possibly not.

KEEPING IT BRIEF

I have a pathological hatred of long-winded email exchanges. In particular, the ones where those involved use the medium as a means to vent; score points; copy in the world and/or complicate an argument.

You may, or may not share my views on this matter.

You may actually be willing to admit that you are 'guilty as charged' of crimes against the keyboard.

I have yet to meet a healthcare manager who isn't inundated with emails. And whilst some of these are essential, my challenge to you is to see if you're willing to have a go at being:

- the person who keeps your responses brief, but appropriate

  and

- the person who categorically refuses to indulge in email exchanges that add no value

I once pondered on the subject of how many hours of UK health service time could be saved by all managers refusing to indulge in unnecessary email conversations. I dare to suggest it might run into millions of hours a year.

So.

Pick a work day when you are going to be tackling some email.

As you work through the messages, make a conscious effort to keep your responses as brief as you can and to sensitively close down any e-dialogue that is in danger of running away with itself.

This doesn't mean being rude, of course. Friendly but factual should work in most cases.

Consciously closing down pointless e-mail exchanges may result in a little more human interaction (help!) – but I promise you this is so much more healthy than hiding behind QWERTY at every opportunity.

Note how differently this approach feels to you and the benefits you gain in respect of working relationships and time saved.

ACKNOWLEDGEMENTS

This book is dedicated to Dan who has been reminding me to 'write it all down' for longer than I dare to admit. Sorry it took so long. And, by the way, you are a legend! I am also hugely indebted to the numerous managers and leaders that allow me into their lives to challenge them to be the best they can be. And to everyone around me for listening, relentlessly, and supporting me in everything I do. If I single you out I will miss someone. So suffice to say, to my twig, my squids and my squad 'I am me because you are you'.

GET IN TOUCH

Skill, will and a healthy dose of courage is the first in a series of guides and workbooks being developed to support managers and clinical leaders. Your feedback, stories and reflections would be most welcome, so please feel free to message me at htaylor88@hotmail.com

MORE REFLECTIONS

Printed in Great Britain
by Amazon

67202899R00081